I0840065

Natural Virus Protection
To Fight Covid-19

Natural Virus Protection
To Fight Covid 19

Improving your Natural Immunity
To the 2020 Coronavirus

by Marlys J. Waters, editor

Power of the Pen Publishing
Nemaha, Iowa

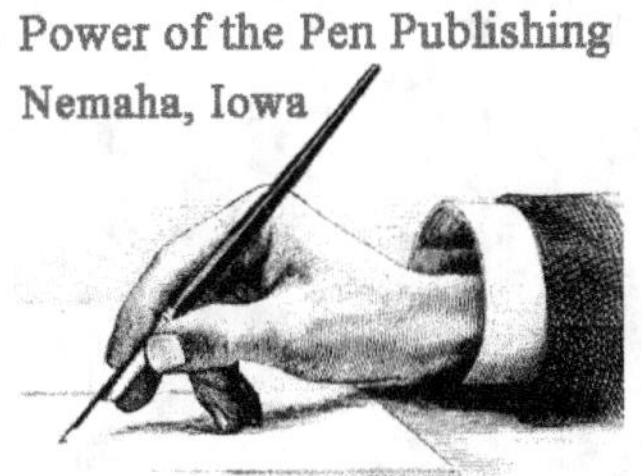

ISBN-13: 978-1-71668-734-1

Published by:
Power of the Pen Publishing
PO Box 5
Nemaha, IA 50567

Table of Contents

I believe it is important in 2020 to get some out-of-print "do-it-yourself" health books back into circulation for the modern times when we expect physicians to cure everything with a pill, an injection, or an operation.

Some modern medications may cure one ailment but cause something worse. That is why I am republishing books from the past that helped maintain our health when more studies were being done on humans brave enough to try different foods, lifestyles, and exercise rather than current pharmaceutical labs that only work at the molecular level with pills.

Don't get me wrong, the cure for polio, measles, suppression of HIV/AIDS, syphilis, bubonic plague and other scourges of the past have been laid to rest by medical science.

There are now new health disorders that are creeping in which don't seem to respond to previous treatments for viruses, some bacteria, germs, microbes, and other pathogens. Autism is one recent controversial disorder that is still being studied and is not discussed in this book.

With modern genetic testing on the source of our food products, it is always safe to go back to the olden days when you raised your own garden produce without the use of genetically modified seeds and fertilizers that may no longer host the trace vitamins and minerals that are so important to our health.

In other words, don't expect the doctor to cure all your sickness with a pill, a shot, or surgery. Your very health may start at home with a book. Many great minds left behind their knowledge in the form of books. Don't be hesitant to pick up a dusty copy published many years earlier. Brilliant minds may have already invented home cures for other physical disorders.

One further warning: Don't believe everything you hear and read, trust your intuition. There are also some quacks that have written books which can ruin your health.

The Coronavirus - COVID-19 - <u>March 2020</u>

The March, 2020 statistics show the wide spread virus infection in the northern hemisphere called the **Coronavirus or COVID-19**, which is spreading panic across several continents.

This is one (of many) news updates on **March 4, 2020**:

- California reported its first death from COVID-19, in an elderly adult with underlying health conditions, the Sacramento Bee reported. The resident of Placer County had taken a cruise from San Francisco to Mexico Feb. 11 to Feb. 21 and was potentially exposed while abroad.

- Italy's government announced Wednesday all schools and universities in the country will be closed from March 5 to March 15, as the country now has more than 2,500 cases and 79 deaths linked to the coronavirus, CNBC reported.

- Los Angeles County reported six new cases of the novel coronavirus on Wednesday (March 4). All of the cases are linked with an "assumed known exposure," such as a history of travel, exposure to a traveler or close contact with a known case, officials said. The county declared a local health emergency to better prepare for and respond to the virus.

- The global mortality rate for COVID-19 is 3.4%, WHO said on March 2. This virus causes more severe illness than the flu, but doesn't spread as efficiently, <u>the director-general said</u>.

- The Olympic Games, scheduled for this summer in Tokyo, will likely continue as planned but there's a chance it <u>could be postponed</u> until later this year amid the coronavirus outbreak.

- Washington state reported three more deaths from the coronavirus on Tuesday.

- FDA announces 1 million coronavirus tests should be available by end of week.

The Coronavirus - COVID-19 Worldwide July 2020

Disclaimer: National updates are published at different times and in different time zones. This, and the time ECDC needs to process these data, may lead to discrepancies between the national numbers and the numbers published by ECDC. Users are advised to use all data with caution and awareness of their limitations. Data are subject to retrospective corrections; corrected datasets are released as soon as processing of updated national data has been completed.

Since 31 December 2019 and as of 30 July 2020, 17 005 983 cases of COVID-19 (in accordance with the applied case definitions and testing strategies in the affected countries) have been reported, including 666 857 deaths.

Cases have been reported from:

- Africa: 892 116 cases; the five countries reporting most cases are South Africa (471 123), Egypt (93 356), Nigeria (42 208), Ghana (35 142) and Algeria (29 229).
- Asia: 4 062 743 cases; the five countries reporting most cases are India (1 583 792), Iran (298 909), Pakistan (277 402), Saudi Arabia (272 590) and Bangladesh (232 194).
- America: 9 169 607 cases; the five countries reporting most cases are United States (4 426 982), Brazil (2 552 265), Mexico (408 449), Peru (400 683) and Chile (351 575).
- Europe: 2 863 459 cases; the five countries reporting most cases are Russia (828 990), United Kingdom (301 455), Spain (282 641), Italy (246 776) and Germany (206 926).
- Oceania: 17 362 cases; the five countries reporting most cases are Australia (15 582), New Zealand (1 210), Guam (354), Papua New Guinea (63) and French Polynesia (62).
- Other: 696 cases have been reported from an international conveyance in Japan.
- Deaths have been reported from:

- Africa: 18 857 deaths; the five countries reporting most deaths are South Africa (7 497), Egypt (4 728), Algeria (1 186), Nigeria (873) and Sudan (725).
- Asia: 92 853 deaths; the five countries reporting most deaths are India (34 968), Iran (16 343), Pakistan (5 924), Turkey (5 659) and Indonesia (4 975).
- America: 351 391 deaths; the five countries reporting most deaths are United States (150 713), Brazil (90 134), Mexico (45 361), Peru (18 816) and Colombia (9 454).
- Europe: 203 542 deaths; the five countries reporting most deaths are United Kingdom (45 961), Italy (35 129), France (30 238), Spain (28 441) and Russia (13 673).
- Oceania: 207 deaths; the 5 countries reporting deaths are Australia (176), New Zealand (22), Guam (5), Northern Mariana Islands (2) and Papua New Guinea (2).
- Other: 7 deaths have been reported from an international conveyance in Japan.
- NOTE: On 17 July 2020, Kyrgyzstan has changed their registration statistics on COVID-19 by introducing two codes (laboratory confirmed cases and clinical-epidemiological cases). This leads to a significant increase in case and death numbers on 18 July 2020.

Is there a reason to panic? Not if you understand that this is just one more of many viruses that threaten the northern hemisphere every winter. However, this one is much more deadly and contagious than when we normally see in the United States winters that didn't even slow down during the hot summer of 2020.

So should we stop mixing with other people, close all the schools, churches, quit traveling, lock up all small businesses? NO! Humans who are healthy will not become infected with the virus if they know how to keep their system healthy. A healthy human body fights daily against invading germs, virus, common colds and much more.

Our eating habits are what are lowering our resistance to infections and other health disorders. Surprisingly the solution is very simple and has been around for years.

The Importance of a Healthy Immune System is for fighting foreign invaders in the body, like pathogenic bacteria and viruses. It can also destroy cells within the body when they have become cancerous.

Poor nutrition results in increased infections, slow healing from injury and infections, and increases susceptibility to complications from immune system dysfunction.

Studies shows that immune function often decreases with age, and recent research suggests this decrease is also related to nutrition and may be slowed or even stopped by maintaining healthy nutrition. However not everyone will take the time to study and practice eating healthy to keep their PH in balance. It is the rest of us that can avoid getting sick just by taking good care of our nutrient intake and give up on the foods/beverages and lifestyles that contribute to lowered immune systems that pick up all the bugs that we encounter. Read on for the 3 simple recommendations to boost your natural immunity immediately.

This section originated from recommendations of Integrative Medicine by Dr. Taz. With the current Coronavirus crisis, having a strong immune system to fight illness is more important than ever.

So how do you boost immunity? By eating the right foods and avoiding the wrong ones. Here are 6 simple steps to reclaiming your immunity:

#1: Start Your Morning with a Tablespoon of apple cider vinegar (ACV) in a cup of water. This will keep your pH balanced. The pH scale in our bodies ranges from 1 to 14, with 7.3 to 7.45 being our ideal range, and can be determined by using a saliva or urine test. If it is Lower than 7.3, you are two acidic and are more likely to have a weak immune system; higher than 7.45, you're too alkaline and could have trouble metabolizing key nutrients, or have low oxygen levels in the blood.

A small amount of ACV (1 tablespoon) diluted in a cup of water twice a day is ample for improving immunity. It helps with gut health by improving the gut microbiome and helping with the metabolism of fat which help keep your immunity healthy.

#2 Drink a Daily Immune Booster. When I think of building an immune system, I focus on increasing your cellular oxygen. levels to fight off viruses and bacteria, beating inflammation, and building up essential nutrients. One beneficial and popular tea is Turmeric Pepper Honey Tea. Black or green tea both are known to help the body fight viruses. Turmeric, is known to fight inflammation and balance hormones.

Black pepper, also an anti-inflammatory, boosts turmeric's bioavailability (you get more bang for your buck); and honey is one of nature's immunity building agents.

#3: Eat to Heal Your Adrenals. You have two adrenal glands, one on top of each of your kidneys. Your adrenals are responsible for producing your stress hormones. Keeping them in check will keep your immunity maximized because chronic stress is one of the hardest blows your immune system can experience.

The key to adrenal balance and health? Eating every 3 to 4 hours, and getting 60 grams of protein a day – that is 15 to 20 grams a meal and 7 to 10 grams at snacks.

Plain Greek yogurt, chicken, fish, are your best choices, and (as long as red meat doesn't cause you digestive problems) include some grass-fed beef or lamb a couple of times a week.

#4: Bulk Up on Magnesium. Have a daily dose of leafy greens such as **spinach**, kale, Swiss chard, or beet greens. These are highest in magnesium. Almonds are also high in magnesium.

I call magnesium the miracle micronutrient because it works as a cofactor for hormones and neurotransmitters, and it is also calming, relaxing, promotes sleep and reduces anxiety. Being overly-stressed and sleep-deprived makes you more susceptible to getting sick. Enjoy them steamed with a teaspoon of olive oil and seasoned

with salt and pepper.

#5: Include Probiotic Foods. These good bacteria are important in balancing your gut (which balances your hormones). A healthy gut supports a healthy immune system.

They are naturally found in certain foods such as yogurt, kefir, bone broth, sourdough bread, and kombucha. Aim to have a serving or two of these foods daily.

#6: Avoid Inflammation-Causing Culprits. Inflammation is an immune response that happens when your body perceives a threat. Highly processed foods, refined, sugars and carbohydrates, red, fatty meats, and alcohol are the top offenders.

Also many people have found that gluten, lactose, and dairy foods can set off inflammation because these foods can disrupt or damage digestion. When the gut is damaged or hindered, it literally switches on an inflammatory cascade that puts your body on the defensive, which then affects your hormone balance and production.

#7 Drink a Daily Immune Booster. When I think of building an immune system, I focus on increasing your cellular oxygen levels to fight off viruses and bacteria, beating inflammation, and building up essential nutrients.

The main recommendation is Turmeric Pepper Honey Tea. Black or green tea both are known to help the body fight viruses. Turmeric, is known to fight inflammation and balance hormones..

Black pepper is also an anti-inflammatory which boosts turmeric's bioavailability (you get more bang for your buck). Also honey is one of nature's immunity building agents.

#8: Eat to Heal Your Adrenals. You have two adrenal glands, one on top of each of your kidneys. Your adrenals are responsible for producing your stress hormones, and keeping them in check. They will then keep your immunity maximized because chronic stress is one of the hardest blows your immune system can experience.

#9:The key to adrenal balance and health? Eating every 3 to 4 hours, and getting 60 grams of protein a day (or 15 to 20 grams a meal and 7 to 10 grams at snacks.) Plain Greek yogurt, chicken and fish, are your best choices. If red meat doesn't cause you digestive problems, you can include some grass-fed beef or lamb a couple of times a week.

End of recommendations by Dr. Taz.

How the healthy human body fights against invasion of dangerous microorganisms.

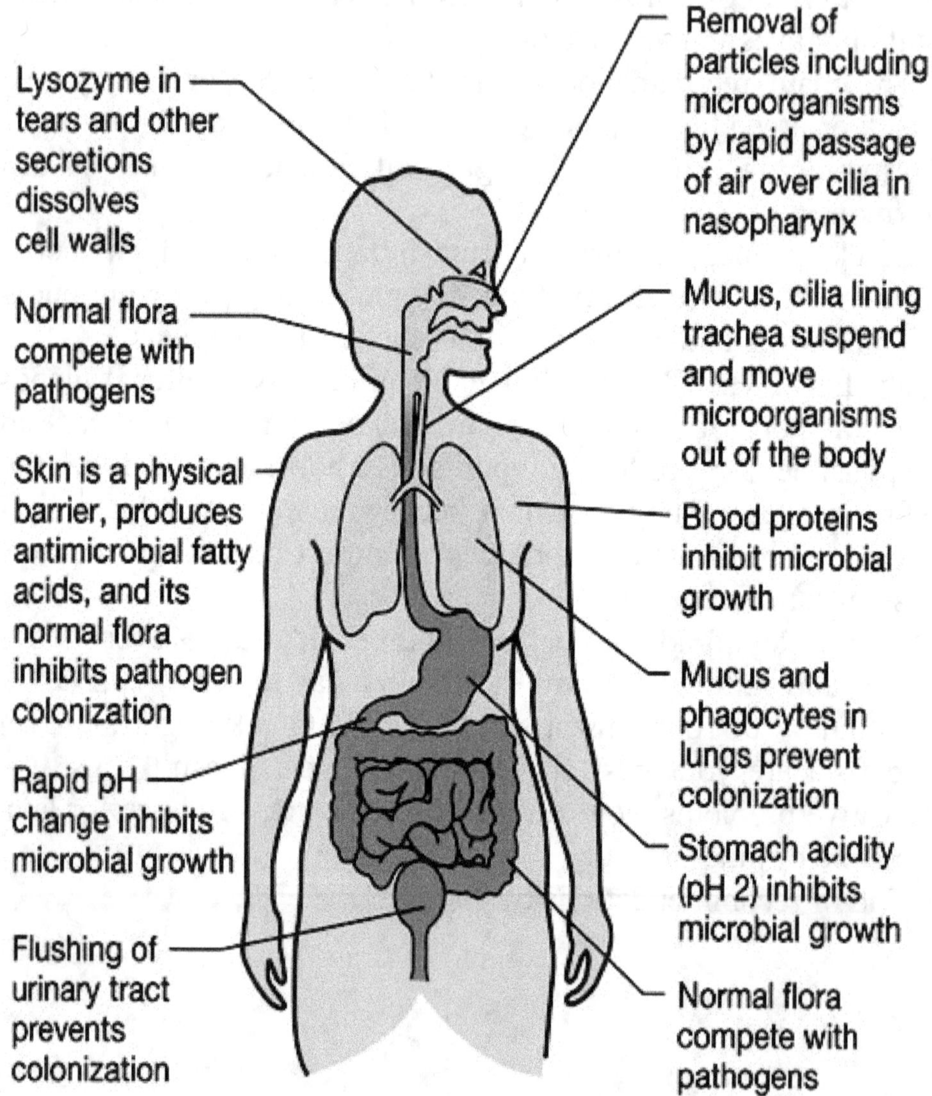

So if the human body has all this natural immunity against disease, virus, and other microorganisms, why do we get sick anyway?

It is because we are eating unhealthy foods for taste only that are actually interfering with our natural immunity.

A Healthy Body Has Natural Resistance against Disease

The immune system protects the body against disease or other potentially damaging foreign bodies. When functioning properly, the immune system identifies and attacks a variety of threats, including viruses, bacteria and parasites, while distinguishing them from the body's own healthy tissue.

The Lymphatic system consists of bone marrow, spleen, thymus and lymph nodes.

- Bone marrow produces white blood cells, or leukocytes.
- The spleen - the largest lymphatic organ in the body, contains white blood cells that fight infection or disease.
- The thymus is where T-cells mature. T-cells help destroy infected or cancerous cells.
- Lymph nodes produce and store cells that fight infection and disease.
- Lymphocytes and leukocytes are small white blood cells that play a large role in defending the body against disease.
- The two types of lymphocytes are B-cells, which make antibodies that attack bacteria and toxins, and T-cells, which help destroy infected or cancerous cells.
- Leukocytes are white blood cells that identify and eliminate pathogens .

The first thing you need to give up is white sugar – the highly processed treat we have all grown to love and that has become a major staple in most all meals. It is often added by the diner as a syrup, sprinkles, frostings, or eaten in ice cream, candy, cookies, cakes, and other favorite sweets.

Sugar gives you lots of quick (but short-lived) energy, and gives you a feel-good feeling for a little while. Yet that sugar is attacking your body and will be explained more in this book.

A healthy body tests slightly acidic and is able to fight off infections. One that is overly alkaline is sick and unable to heal as the tissues, organs, skin, blood in the arteries and vessels, and even the brain will start to deteriorate.

However, a system can be TOO acidic. Being too acidic is not suitable for your body. This condition may conceive various symptoms which cause you to suffer from them. You may think you have harmful diseases, and you have a weak immune system, etc. But probably the main reason for all of these is just too acidic. Therefore, you need to check the list of symptoms of being too acidic and start a more alkaline diet.

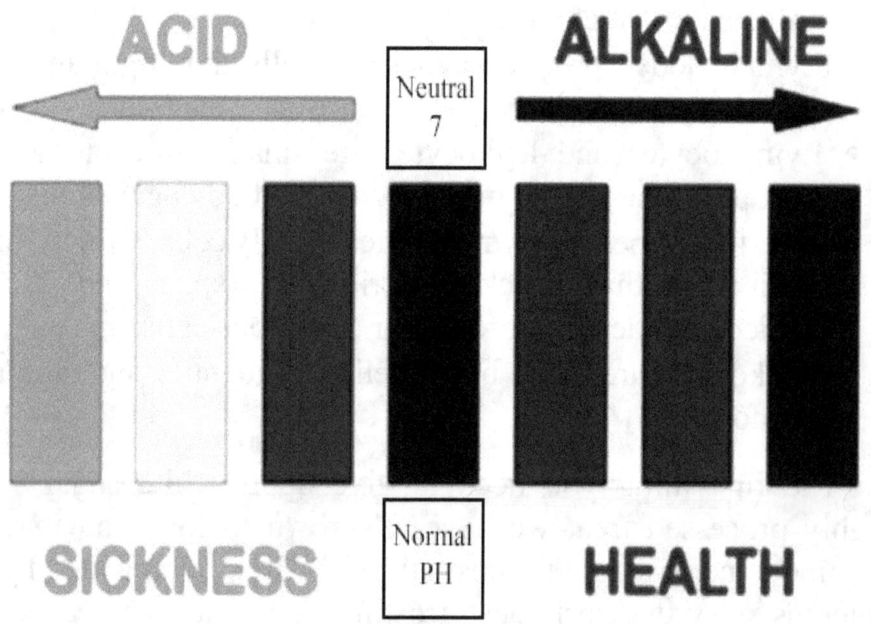

Controlling Acidic and Alkaline PH

Follows is the list of symptoms of being too acidic:

Having Unhealthy Skin

Having unhealthy skin is just one of the symptoms of being too acidic. If your nails are thin and you complain that they break easily, the restorative, over-the-counter cosmetics can't help you. Plus, you may have dry skin, and your lips' corners may crack. Again cosmetics can't solve this. Being too acidic can also cause your hair to thin and fall out.

Having Unhealthy Mouth and Teeth

Being too acidic can cause not only sensitive teeth but also losing your teeth. You may notice tooth pain and sensitive gums which may be a signal of infection eating away the base of your teeth.

Having Digestive Problems

Lots of people suffer from digestive problems when eating too much sugar. Being too acidic from any cause makes digestion harder which can result in acid reflux, ulcers, and gastritis.

Being Joyless and Depressed

If you feel like you're depressed and your experience with drugs to alleviate depression are useless, try to think about acidic foods as a possible cause. They tend to lower your energy and suppress joy and bliss. You may also may nervous for no reason.

Being Too Acidic Affects Your Whole Body

If you usually consume excessive acidic foods, you may tend to have headaches, leg cramps, and eye infection (conjunctivitis), This condition affects not only your metabolism but your eye health too. Having a low body temperature is another symptom. If you get frequent infections, it may be because your body is too acidic due to your eating habits.

How to avoid being too acidic.

The path to an alkaline lifestyle is not difficult. By keeping the ratio of acidic food at around 30% and alkaline diet at approximately 70% will do the trick.. Suggestions follow:

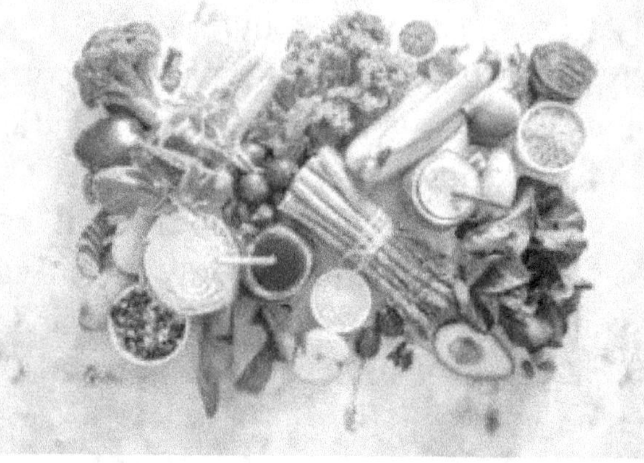

1. Go green

Vegetables, some fruits, seeds, nuts, and roots are naturally alkalizing. Increasing the amount of these in your diet will help reduce your consumption of acidic foods like meat or grains.

Avocados, beetroot (the root portion of the beet plant), spinach, kale (if you have access to it which is at the top of the recommended nutrition/calorie chart), and cucumbers which also help boost your alkalinity.

2. Consume less acidic foods

It is challenging to cut out the naturally addictive foods such as meat, eggs, processed sugars, flour, and dairy products that you've grown to love. However, it is easier to reduce their amount in your daily diet to less than 30% which is a good start.

3. Limit alcohol consumption

Alcohol may cause different issues in our lives. However, it inevitably causes dietary problems due to very high sugar content. An occasional glass of wine or a few beers while enjoying a sports game is acceptable for social benefit. However, alcohol should be consumed responsibly. Otherwise, it makes the body acidic very quickly.

4. Drinking alkaline water

Most of us do not drink enough water. Everyone should drink up to 8 large glasses of water every day, preferably alkaline water since it has a higher pH level than tap water. "7" is a neutral pH. The higher the pH level the more alkaline, or basic, it is. The lower the pH level, the more acidic it is. Tap water and bottled water have a pH of up to 7. Alkaline water has an average pH of 9 which helps at balancing the alkaline-acid levels in the body. Don't worry if finding alkaline water is not available. Just keep drinking tap water (treated and tested for humans) and you'll be fine.

5. Choose drinks carefully

Caffeine-containing drinks such as coffee, some teas, and energy drinks often create a craving for sugar to suppress "the shakes" and/or inability to fall asleep in those who do not tolerate caffeine well. Choosing natural, alkalizing drinks such as herbal teas, lemon water and caffeine/free teas can help cleanse the digestive system, optimize metabolism and eradicate excess acid.

Seven things you should know about the Coronavirus
This section was written by a registered nurse in 2020.

1. Coronavirus itself isn't new. Just like influenza, coronavirus is a family of respiratory viruses, and there are multiple strains, which have the ability to change over time. Coronavirus is already common in the United States, and has been for years. I have personally cared for patients with this diagnosis.

2. Novel coronavirus, also known as COVID-19, is the strain we're hearing about in the news. It emerged in Wuhan, China at the end of 2019.

3. Symptoms of COVID-19 include fever, cough, and shortness of breath. Just like the flu and common cold, it is spread person to person via respiratory droplets when an infected person coughs or sneezes.

4. According to the World Health Organization, as of <u>February 26, 2020</u>, there have been 2,918 confirmed cases of COVID-19 outside of China. 53 of these are in the United States. There have been 44 deaths, none in the United States. Compare this to influenza, which the CDC estimates will infect between 29,000,000 and 41,000,000 people in the United States alone during the 2019-20 season, resulting in 16,000 to 41,000 deaths.

5. So far in July of 2020, there is no cure!" There's no magic pill that cures the common flu either. But there is a flu vaccine (that doesn't cause autism) that can protect you from our most common respiratory viruses. Maybe it may improve your immunity to the Coronavirus while not actually guaranteeing 100% immunity. If you are symptom free and haven't had a yearly flu shot, you may improve your chances of immunity to COVID-19 by getting a flu shot ASAP.

6. So, why are we panicking? Frankly because the media tells us to. Manufacturing a pandemic is a great way to boost ratings, but everything science knows so far about COVID-19 has revealed it to be just another respiratory virus (and there are thousands) until it starting spreading fast and creating not only a

significant percentage of deaths but also continuing disorders lingering after recovery for those who survived..

7. The scariest part of COVID-19 isn't the virus itself, it's the resulting mass paranoia. Hospitals are hoarding supplies, creating shortages of PPE (personal protective equipment) necessary to protect healthcare workers and patients. Cities are refusing to house and treat sick people who have nowhere else to go. People are using the virus as an excuse for their own social prejudices.

So, what can you do? Turn off the TV and arm yourself with the facts. Stop the spread of false information.

And for Pete's sake, wash your hands.

(Information & statistics obtained directly from the CDC & WHO TV)

Benefits of Apple Cider Vinegar

Editor's Warnings:

1) Apple Cider <u>Flavored</u> vinegar is NOT the same thing as pure Apple Cider Vinegar.

2) <u>White Vinegar</u> is NOT the same as Pure Apple Cider Vinegar. Normally any bottle that lists the contents as "Apple Cider Vinegar" with no other wording IS the right solution.

3) A dose of 1 teaspoon of Apple Cider Vinegar is all that is necessary to correct a temporary PH imbalance and may safely be taken twice a day in water or fruit/vegetable juice. A capful (lid from the bottle) is equal to 1 teaspoon so you don't need any special measuring equipment.

It should not be taken with medications. ACV is quickly digested through the stomach so can be taken ½ hour before or ½ hour after scheduled medications. ACV should also not be taken without a liquid to wash it down. When it reaches the stomach acidity it is harmless and does its work along with normal stomach acids to help digest food and is absorbed through the circulatory system (blood) to clear out plaque and disable and destroy any virus that are invading your body.

If you drink Apple Cider Vinegar without a cushioning liquid like water or juice, it may irritate your throat and pit your teeth. The stomach can handle acid which it creates on its own to digest your food.

Also DO NOT <u>overindulge</u> in Apple Cider Vinegar. Too much can worsen your Acid/Alkaline imbalance and aggravate any conditions you are already dealing with. I know one man who decided to drink a cup of Apple Cider Vinegar even though he had been told to use no more than 1 teaspoon twice a day in water or other liquid. He got a major belly ache that night and realized how dangerous an overdose can be and which can even lead to stomach ulcers.

Apple cider vinegar has been around for a long time. Its use dates back thousands of years. It's been used for detoxification, treating pneumonia, and even assisting with weight loss. Some claim that the ancient Greek physician Hippocrates used it to cure a host of ailments.

This book is concerned with helping control a healthy PH balance to improve your chances of avoiding invading virus and other unhealthy microorganisms so little discussion will be delivered on assisting with a weight loss program.

.**End of Author's Warnings**.

The balance of discussion on Apple Cider Vinegar has been taken from the book "Vermont Folk Medicine" by Dr. D. C. Jarvis, originally published in 1958 and still available online from various book sellers.

How does Apple Cider Vinegar work?

So how does apple cider vinegar help people become resistant to virus infections, common colds, bronchitis, etc? It accelerates the body's ability to break down and derive nutrients from fats and protein efficiently and quickly from the digestive system, which means a faster metabolism and more vitality to fight internal germs and virus looking for a tolerable and accepting host to multiply. A body with a PH imbalance is a welcome place for germs, virus, and other diseases/disorders to multiply.

Additional benefits of Apple Cider Vinegar

While vinegar seems to have an acidic quality to it, it actually does just the opposite in your body. "Apple cider vinegar helps the body maintain an alkaline pH, which is widely regarded as anti-cancer and promotes general vitality and wellbeing," says Jansen.

Your body's pH is a measure of your body's acidity and alkalinity. Severe acidity can lead to a number of health problems, like acidosis which affects the kidneys, lungs and resulting kidney stones.

Keeping your alkaline pH balanced is essential for maintaining good health. Severe acidity can lead to a number of health problems, like acidosis and kidney stones.

Apple cider vinegar as a supplement or applied topically can also be good for the skin. When applied topically, it regulates the pH of the skin and has a great effect fighting age spots, acne, and even warts, "It has a detoxifying effect on the liver which will show up in a glowing healthy complexion. Its beneficial bacteria will contribute to healthy skin as well, because our skin is a reflection of what is inside us as well as what is outside us."

Reminder

People who intend to use apple cider vinegar should ensure that it is heavily diluted. Normal dosage is 1 teaspoon of Apple Cider Vinegar diluted with a cup of water, V8 juice or other natural juice is the safest. "Make sure you rinse your mouth with clear water afterwards, as the cider vinegar can pit the teeth if not rinsed off.

A teaspoon of Apple Cider Vinegar with a cup of liquid (water, juice) should be taken on an empty stomach and is promptly digested and absorbed into the circulatory system (blood) where it does its work eliminating virus, thinning blood clots, and more.

Apple Cider Vinegar even comes in pills/tablets. Just keep in mind that to digest a pill or tablet takes longer than drinking the liquid which is absorbed into your blood stream through the stomach much faster to do its work. I've not read any tests on the benefits or disadvantages of ACV pills.

Author does not endorse any particular brand. I've used the following over the years and have not noticed any significant difference in results other than they all seem to work equally well at keeping virus, flu and colds at bay.

Types of Apple Cider Vinegar

1. Filtered Apple Cider Vinegar is a clear light gold color with a milder apple flavor. It is commonly cheaper that unfiltered.

2. Unfiltered apple cider vinegar has traces of the mother which may hold health benefits and allows you to make your own vinegar with it. Unfiltered brands consist of strands of proteins, enzymes, and friendly bacteria that give the product a murky appearance "Organic" Apple Cider Vinegar is often associated with the unfiltered brands which go through the same process without filtering.

Apple Cider vinegars are 5–6% acetic acid.

Apple cider vinegar has other health benefits which will not be included in this book which is primarily dealing with virus protection.

However I will mention that it may have appetite-suppressing effects, having been shown to slow the rate at which food leaves your stomach which is why it is recommended you not take it with food or medications.

Author only uses 1 teaspoon or about a bottle cap full mixed in a cup of water or V8 juice, (not a tablespoon full as some recommend). When in doubt use the smaller amount.

Steps to Achieve a healthy PH-balance – from Healthline

Your body's pH balance, also referred to as its acid-base balance, is the level of acids and bases in your blood at which your body functions best. A normal blood pH level is 7.40 on a scale of 0 to 14, where 0 is the most acidic and 14 is the most basic.

This value can vary slightly in either direction. Fortunately, making your organism more alkaline is simple and is the opposite of acidic environment.

Here are 10 simple natural ways that you can practice every day to alkalize your organism. You will soon gain more everyday energy and vitality:

1) The most important thing is to start your day with a large glass of water with the juice of a freshly-squeezed lemon. Lemons actually have the opposite effect on your body even they may seem acidic. Drink first thing in the morning to flush the system.

2) Another option is to drink one or two glasses of water with organic apple cider vinegar. You should dilute one tablespoons of pure apple cider vinegar in eight ounces of water.

3) Eat a large portion of green salad tossed in lemon juice and quality olive oil. Greens (vegetable or fruit) are among the best sources of alkaline minerals, like calcium. Eat alkaline foods during the day like fruits and vegetables. They sustain the body's pH on a daily basis and keep balance in your organism.

4) Your snack should consist on raw, unsalted almonds. Almonds are full of minerals that are natural alkaline like magnesium and calcium, which actually help to balance out acidity and at the same time to balance blood sugar.

5) Drink almond milk and make yourself a berry smoothie with added green powder like spirulina, or other greens. If

you have choice between almond milk and cow's milk, almond milk is a better option.

6) Go for a walk or some other exercise. It's very important to be active. Exercise actually helps move acidic products so your body can better eliminate them.

7) Breathe deeply. Ideally choose a spot that has fresh, oxygen-rich air and go there whenever you can. If you live in a city with tall buildings and lots of automobile traffic, you may need to find a quiet side-street where there would be fresher air not filled with auto exhaust fumes. Continue to drink lots of water on a daily basis to flush the system of waste.

8) Do not eat meat every day. If you can skip a few days without meat it will help get rid of excess acid. Eating meat every day leaves an acid residue behind. On non-meat days you can select vegan or vegetarian entrees to help Alkalize your body!

9) Add more vegetables to your diet. Be careful, white potatoes count as a starch. However, sweet potatoes are a good choice, just don't make them with butter. Use olive oil for baking. Peppers. Asparagus squash, and other vegetables are also great choices.

10) And last but not least: Add more sprouts to your daily diet. They are extremely alkalizing and rich in nutrients and energy-boosting enzymes.

11) Skip desserts loaded with sugar and skip drinking soda beverages that are sweetened with sugar. is one of the worst acidic foods we consume. If you drink just ONE can of soda with sugar, you will actually need more than thirty glasses of neutral water to neutralize the acidity in your body! A person can survive with better health if they omit all pure sugars from their diet.

The Four Sugars

This chapter is optional reading. It merely gives more details on types of sugar and artificial sugars. If you are already convinced that sugar in any form is not good for the human body, you may skip this chapter.

Glucose is the sugar in blood, and **dextrose** is the name given to glucose produced from corn. Biochemically they are identical.

Fructose is the principal sugar in fruit. It raises no issues in fruit because it is accompanied by nutrients and fiber.

Sucrose is table sugar. It is a double sugar, containing one part each of glucose (50%) and fructose (50%), chemically bound together. Enzymes in the intestine quickly and efficiently split sucrose into glucose and fructose, which are absorbed into the body as single sugars.

High Fructose Corn Syrup or HFCS is made from corn starch. It contains roughly equivalent amounts of glucose (45 to 58%) and fructose (42 to 55%). HFCS raises several issues, <u>health</u> and otherwise:

Concerns about High Fructose Corn Syrup

U S Americans (all ages) consume about 60 pounds of sucrose and <u>another 60 pounds of HFCS each year</u>. This is way more than is good for health. Sugars of any kind provide calories but **NO** nutrients.

Increasing evidence suggests that the metabolism of Fructose which differs from that of glucose is associated with abnormalities. This means that it is best to reduce intake of fructose from table sugar as well as HFCS.

There is no reason to study or memorize the following Sugar chart in the next chapter. Basically sugar is a non-food (unless it is part of a healthy fruit) and does little good but causes damage in the human body. You will be more susceptible to colds, flu and other virus infections, diabetes, heart disease, and even kidney failure if you add lots of sugar to your diet.

Table of Sugar Comparisons of Human Tolerance

Sugar	Description	HFI Tolerance
Agave Syrup	From the blue agave cactus. Commonly used in Tex-Mex foods, tequila, margaritas, soft drinks. High in fructose.	Not Tolerated
Aspartame	Sugar substitute known as Equal, NutraSweet, NutraTase. FDA approved. Scientifically studied in depth. Some may be sensitive to headaches.Derived from amino acids.	Tolerated
Acesulfame-K	Sugar substitute known as Sunette, SwissSweet, Sweet-One. Was approved by FDA, but Center for Science in the Public Interest (CSPI) recently questioned safety. Possible carcinogenic.	Tolerated (Questionable safety)
Baker's Sugar	Another name for Bar Sugar, Berry Sugar, Castor/Caster sugar, Ultrafine,Superfine. Sucrose, Finest of all granulated sugar.	Not Tolerated
Bar Sugar	Another name for Baker's Sugar, Berry Sugar, Castor/Caster sugar, Ultrafine, Superfine. Sucrose, Finest of all granulated sugar.	Not Tolerated
Barbados Sugar	British specialty brown sugar with strong molasses flavor.	Not Tolerated
Barley Malt Syrup	From sprouted grains of barley, kiln dried and cooked with water.	Tolerated
Beet Sugar	Sucrose. Same structure as cane sugar, but may produce different product results because of .05 differences in minerals and proteins. More common in Europe than the U.S	Not Tolerated

Berry Sugar	Another name for Baker's Sugar, Bar Sugar, Castor/Caster sugar, Ultrafine, Superfine. Sucrose. Finest of all granulated sugar.	Not Tolerated
Birch Sugar	Sugar alcohol: Xylitol. Trade name; The Ultimate Sweetener. Derived from xylose.	Tolerated depending on purity
Brown Rice Syrup	Made from brown rice. High protein content. Likely contains sucrose.	Not Tolerated
Brown Sugar	Sucrose coated with molasses.¬Ý	Not Tolerated
Cane Sugar	Sucrose. Table sugar.	Not Tolerated
Castor/Caster Sugar	Another name for Baker's Sugar, Bar Sugar, Berry Sugar, Superfine, Ultrafine. Sucrose. Finest of all granulated sugar.	Not Tolerated
Carob Powder	75% sucrose, pluse glucose and fructose. Extract of the carob tree.	Not Tolerated
Chicory	Contains inulin. Used to make fructose syrup.	Not Tolerated
Chinese Rock Sugar	Combination of honey and sugars.	Not Tolerated
Corn Starch	Derived from corn. Composed of straight or branched chains of glucose.	Tolerated
Corn Sugar	Produced from corn starch. Contains glucose and maltose molecules.	Tolerated
Corn Syrup	Glucose and water. Usually produced from cornstarch. The problem is that in making the syrup, it may have either maltose and/or fructose added.	Not Tolerated
Corn Syrup Solids	Dried glucose syrup.	Caution, needs further clarification
Confectioners Sugar	Sucrose. A chemical combination of glucose and fructose.	Not Tolerated

Date Sugar	Made from dried, pulverized dates. Likely contains sucrose.	Not Tolerated
Demerara	Sucrose. Another name for raw sugar. A chemical combination of glucose and fructose.	Not Tolerated
Dextrin	Glucose molecules linked together in chains. Does not break down to pure dextrose.	Tolerated
Dextrose	Single glucose molecule. Simple sugar.	Tolerated
Dextroglucose	Single glucose molecule. Simple sugar.	Tolerated
Dextrose Monohydrat	Pure dextrose.	Tolerated
D-Allose	Simple sugar.Not commonly found in diet.Made of 6 carbons.	Tolerated
D-Altrose	Simple sugar.Not commonly found in diet.Made of 6 carbons.	Tolerated
D-Arabinose	Simple sugar.Not commonly found in diet.Made of 5 carbons.	Tolerated
D-Erythrose	Simple sugar.Not commonly found in diet.Made of 4 carbons.	Tolerated
D-Erythrulose	Simple sugar.Not commonly found in diet.Made of 4 carbons.	Tolerated¬Ý
D-Galactose	Simple sugar.Not commonly found in diet as free galactose.Made of 6 carbons.¬ÝPart of lactose.	Tolerated¬Ý
D-Gulose	Simple sugar.Not commonly found in diet.Made of 6 carbons.	Tolerated
D-Idose	Simple sugar.Not commonly found in diet.Made of 6 carbons.	Tolerated
D-Lyxose	Simple sugar.Not commonly found in diet.Made of 5 carbons.	Tolerated
D-Psicose	Sweetener.¬ÝMay cause diarrhea. Chemically related to	Tolerated depending on

	fructose.Made of 6 carbons.	purity
D-Ribose	Simple sugar.Not commonly found in diet.Made of 5 carbons.	Tolerated
D-Ribulose	Simple sugar.Not commonly found in diet.Made of 5 carbons.	Tolerated
D-Sorbose	Sweetener.May cause diarrhea. Chemically related to fructose.Made of 6 carbons.	Tolerated depending on purity
D-Tagatose	Sweetener.¬ÝMay cause diarrhea. Chemically related to fructose.Made of 6 carbons.	Tolerated depending on purity
D-Talose	Simple sugar.Not commonly found in diet.Made of 6 carbons.	Tolerated
D-Threose	Simple sugar.Not commonly found in diet.Made of 4 carbons.	Tolerated
D-Xylose	Simple sugar.Not commonly found.Made of 5 carbons.	Tolerated
D-Xyulose	Simple sugar.Not commonly found in diet.Made of 5 carbons.	Tolerated
Dulcitol	Naturally occurring sugar alcohol.	Not Tolerated
Erythitol	Sugar alcohol. Related to erythrose.	Tolerated depending on purity
Evaporated Cane Sug	Sucrose. Another name for sugar cane juice.	Not Tolerated
Fructose	Simple sugar of fructose molecules. Sometimes called fruit sugar.Made of 6 carbons.	Not Tolerated
Fruit Juice Sweetene	Derived from grapes, apples or pears, heated to reduce water leaving a sweeter moreconcentrated juice.Almost pure fructose.	Not Tolerated
Gemsugar	Colored sugar made from Thai sugarcane infused with herbs.	Not Tolerated

Glucose	Simple sugar. The chemical sugar structure of blood sugar.Made of 6 carbons.	Tolerated
Glucose Polymers	Chains of glucose molecules.	Tolerated
Glucose Syrups	Produced from starch, corn syrup, corn-syrup solids, starch syrup, and sugar cane syrup. Another name for glucose.	Caution, needs further clarification
Grape Syrup	Pure fructose.	Not Tolerated
Granulated sugar	Table sugar. Sucrose.¬Ý	Not Tolerated
Gur	Another name for Jaggery. 35% sucrose, 15% reducing sugar (mixture of glucose plus fructose). Used in Thai cooking. Made from palm dates or sugar cane juice. Contains molasses.	Not Tolerated
High Fructose Corn S	Enzymetically converted from corn syrup to contain 42% - 90% fructose. Raises triglyceride levels and increases risk of heart disease.	Not Tolerated
High Fructose glucos	Contains fructose.	Not Tolerated
Honey¬Ý	Natural syrup containing about 35% glucose, 40% fructose, 25 % water	Not Tolerated
Hydrogenated Starch	Sugar alcohol of glucose.	Tolerated depending on purity
Invert Sugar	Created by combining sugar syrup with cream of tarter or lemon juice and heating, breaking sucrose down to components glucose and fructose.	Not Tolerated
Isoglucose	Another name for High Fructose Corn Syrup (HFCS).	Not Tolerated
Isomaltose	Linked glucose molecules that rapidly break down to glucose in the intestine.	Tolerated

Jaggery	Made from either evaporating fresh juice of palm trees, or sugar cane juice. 35% sucrose, 15% reducing sugar (mixture of glucose plus fructose). Contains molasses.	Not Tolerated
Lactitol	Sugar alcohol form of lactose.	Tolerated depending on purity
Lactose	Milk sugar, making up 4.5% of cow's milk. Restricted in lactose intolerant.	Tolerated
Levulose	Contains fructose.	Not Tolerated
Litesse	Polydextrose. Nondigestable polysaccharide. Reduced calorie sugar substitute containing sorbitol and glucose.	Not Tolerated
Maltitol	Sugar alcohol form of maltose (glucose).	Tolerated depending on purity
Maltose	Linked glucose molecules that rapidly break down to glucose in the intestine.¬Ý	Tolerated
Maltodextrin	Dextrose. Processed from natural cornstarch.	Tolerated
Mannitol	Sugar alcohol form of mannose.	Tolerated depending on purity
Mannose	Simple sugar.Not commonly found.	Tolerated
Maple Syrup	Mostly sucrose. Contains some invert sugar.	Not Tolerated
Maple Sugar	Mostly sucrose. Contains some invert sugar.	Not Tolerated
Moducal	Glucose chains. A medical food. Consult physician before use.¬Ý	Tolerated
Molasses	By-product of sugar cane with 24% water. Fructose level varies. Three kinds. Light (sweetest), Medium (darker and less sweet), Blackstrap (very dark, slightly sweet with	Not Tolerated

	distinctive flavor. Good source of calcium and iron)	
Molasses Sugar	Dark muscovado sugar with extra molasses.	Not Tolerated
Muscovado Sugar	Another name for Barbados sugar, a brown sugar with strong molasses flavor.	Not Tolerated
Neotame	Sugar substitute. Synthetic aspartame.	Tolerated
Palm Sugar	Used in Thai cooking. Likely contains sucrose.	Not Tolerated
Panella	35% sucrose, 15% reducing sugar (mixture of glucose plus fructose.) Contains molasses.	Not Tolerated
Polincillo¬Ý	Mexican brown sugar. Semi refined and granulated. No molasses added	Not Tolerated
Polycose	Chains of dextrose. Added to foods to increase calories.	Tolerated
Polydextrin	Chains of glucose molecules. Does not break down to pure dextrose.	Tolerated
Polydextrose	Polydextrose is a multi-purpose additive synthesized from dextrose (glucose), plus about 10 percent sorbitol and 1 percent citric acid. It is commonly used as a replacement for sugar, starch, and fat in commercial cakes, candies, dessert mixes, gelatins, frozen desserts, puddings, and salad dressings.¬ÝSorbitol is a sugar alcohol that is related to fructose.	Not Tolerated
Raffinose	A trisaccharide found in grains, legumes and some vegetables. Gas forming.	Tolerance Varies

Rapadura	35% sucrose, 15% reducing sugar (glucose plus fructose). Contains molasses.	Not Tolerated
Raw Sugar	Sucrose. Equal parts glucose and fructose, a chemical combination of glucose and fructose.	Not Tolerated
Reducing Sugar	Referred to as invert sugar (mixture of glucose and fructose).	Not Tolerated
Rock Sugar	Crystallized cane sugar. Sucrose, a combination of glucose and fructose.	Not Tolerated
Saccharin	Sugar substitute. Not as commonly used as in the past. Known as Sweet N' Low, Sugar Twin, Sucryl, Featherweight. FDA approved. More than 6 servings per day may increase bladder cancer risk. (No longer approved for use in Canada)	Tolerated
Saccharose	Sucrose. Equal parts glucose and fructose.	Not Tolerated
Sorbitol	Sugar alcohol. Common in fruits, particularly skin of ripe berries, cherries and plums. Used in sugar free foods. Causes diarrhea. Converted back to fructose.	Not Tolerated
Splenda	A sugar substitute. This is a chemically modified sucrose molecule that cannnot be digested.	Tolerated depending on purity
Stevia	Natural sweetener from a South American plant. 30 % sweeter than sugar. Used extensively in Japan, China, Korea, Israel, Brazil and Paraguay with no side effects reported. Known as Stevioside. Has not been rigorously tested for safety. No consistent manufacturing regulations.¬Ý	Not Tolerated

Sucanat	Sucrose. Another name for raw sugar. Equal parts glucose and fructose. However, read the labels. Some now listed as Sucanat are cane sugar plus blackstrap molasses.	Not Tolerated
Sucralose	Chemical name for Splenda, a sugar substitute. Large molecule not digested.	Tolerated depending on purity
Sucrose	Naturally occurring sugar made from sugar cane or sugar beets. Commonly referred to as sugar and table sugar. Chemical combination of glucose and fructose.	Not Tolerated
Sucrose Syrups	Also known as Refiner's syrup. By product of sugar refining. 15 ¬Æ¬¢ 18% water, 1 part sucrose to two parts invert sugar.	Not Tolerated
Sugar	Common name for sucrose, a chemical combination of glucose and fructose.	Not Tolerated
Sugar Alcohol	May be naturally or synthetically occurring. Causes diarrhea. This is a reduced form of sugar that may be metabolized back to fructose or other sugars depending on the type.	Not Tolerated
Trimoline	Produced from beets. Up to 22 % invert sugar. 28 % sweeter than granulated sugar	Not Tolerated
Turbinado	Another name for raw sugar. Sucrose, a chemical combination of glucose and fructose.	Not Tolerated
Vanilla sugar	Sucrose. Made by burying vanilla beans in cane sugar for weeks. A chemical combination of glucose and fructose.	Not Tolerated

Wasanbon	Grown on an island in the area of Japan from a special variety of sugar cane. A pale beige powder of very pure sugar. Not good for cooking. Melts immediately on the tongue. Very scarce and very expensive.	Not Tolerated
Xylitol	Sugar alcohol. Obtained from fruits and berries. Also from birch trees and known as birch sugar. Causes diarrhea.	Tolerated depending on purity
Xylose	Simple sugar.Not commonly found.¬ÝMade of 5 carbons.	Tolerated

Artificial Sweeteners Can Lead to Dementia

The artificial sweeteners used in diet sodas and thousands of other processed foods are anything but sweet. In fact, they can be toxic to the brain. Consuming these sugar substitutes on a regular basis is not a recipe for a healthy memory.

Sherry, who weighed over 200 pounds on her 5'5" frame, guzzled diet soda thinking it would help her lose weight. It didn't. Even worse, she started experiencing a host of symptoms—digestive issues, arthritis, forgetfulness, and confusion. In fact, Sherry's diet soda habit was hurting her brain and putting her memory at risk.

That's what a growing body of evidence shows. For example, one study found that drinking diet soda was linked to an increased risk of Alzheimer's disease and other forms of dementia.

Ways Artificial Sweeteners Steal Your Mind

1. Aspartame overstimulates neurotransmitters. One of the most commonly used artificial sweeteners in diet sodas, aspartame is particularly damaging to the brain. Consider how it impacts aspartate, an excitatory neurotransmitter associated with memory as well as learning and pain perception. Aspartame stimulates this neurotransmitter and can damage neurons, cause cell death, and is associated with a host of issues including memory problems and dementia.

2. Artificial sweeteners contribute to chronically high insulin. Elevated insulin levels increase your risk for Alzheimer's disease and also raise the risk of heart disease, diabetes, metabolic syndrome, and other health problems.

3. Artificial sweeteners in diet sodas may lower metabolism. For anyone who thinks diet sodas help with weight loss, the reality is that artificial sweeteners can lead to weight gain. Studies of rats fed artificially sweetened foods showed slower metabolisms and greater weight gain than those given sugar-sweetened foods despite the fact that the rats that ate sugary

The Danger of Artificial Sweeteners and your Mind

Now that you have succeeded in the previous chapter and the dangers of sugar you are now an overview on the dangers of artificial sweeteners.

Artificial Sweeteners Can Lead to Dementia and other Disorders

The artificial sweeteners used in diet sodas and thousands of other processed foods are anything but sweet. In fact, they can be toxic to the brain. Consuming these sugar substitutes on a regular basis is not a recipe for a healthy memory.

Sherry, who weighed over 200 pounds on her 5'5" frame, guzzled diet soda thinking it would help her lose weight. It didn't. Even worse, she started experiencing a host of symptoms—digestive issues, arthritis, forgetfulness, and confusion. In fact, Sherry's diet soda habit was hurting her brain and putting her memory at risk.

That's what a growing body of evidence shows. For example, one study found that drinking diet soda was linked to an increased risk of Alzheimer's disease and other forms of dementia.

Ways Artificial Sweeteners Steal Your Mind

1. Aspartame overstimulates neurotransmitters. One of the most commonly used artificial sweeteners in diet sodas, aspartame is particularly damaging to the brain. Consider how it impacts aspartate, an excitatory neurotransmitter associated with memory as well as learning and pain perception. Aspartame stimulates this neurotransmitter and can damage neurons, cause cell death, and is associated with a host of issues including memory problems and dementia.

2. Artificial sweeteners contribute to chronically high insulin. Elevated insulin levels increase your risk for Alzheimer's disease and also raise the risk of heart disease, diabetes, metabolic syndrome, and other health problems.

3. Artificial sweeteners in diet sodas may lower metabolism. For anyone who thinks diet sodas help with weight loss, the

reality is that artificial sweeteners can lead to weight gain. Studies of rats fed artificially sweetened foods showed slower metabolisms and greater weight gain than those given sugar-sweetened foods despite the fact that the rats that ate sugary foods consumed more calories than those that ate artificially sweetened foods. Both diabetes and obesity are considered independent risk factors for memory problems and several forms of dementia.

4. Artificial sugar substitutes mess with gut health. A 2018 found that six artificial sweeteners (aspartame, sucralose, saccharine, neotame, advantame, and acesulfame potassium-k) had toxic effects on gut bacteria. Compromised gut bacteria can lead to issues such as leaky gut, a condition in which the lining of the gut becomes excessively permeable. Leaky gut has been linked to the development of Alzheimer's disease and other dementias.

Sweeter Alternatives

If you want to avoid sugar and don't want the damage that comes from artificial sweeteners, here are two options.

Erythritol, a sugar alcohol that comes in crystals or powder form, is calorie-free and doesn't cause blood sugar or insulin levels to spike. (Note: Be aware that sugar alcohols, such as Xylitol and Maltitol, may cause GI distress.)

Stevia, a natural plant extract, is 200-300 times sweeter than sugar, but it does not impact blood sugar levels the way sugar does. Some evidence suggests stevia may stabilize blood sugar. However more research is needed. (Note: If you take medication for blood pressure or diabetes, talk to a healthcare provider before using stevia.)

It is critical for any changes in memory or cognitive function to be investigated. Research shows that changes in the brain from Alzheimer's disease can start decades before any symptoms arise. At this stage, there is imaging available to see what is happening in the brain as part of a comprehensive evaluation that also includes cognitive testing and a detailed look at the biological, psychological, social, and spiritual factors that may be contributing to memory issues.

Are Artificial Sweeteners Toxic to the Brain?

As sugar's harmful effects are becoming more widely acknowledged, the consumption of artificially sweetened foods and drinks is increasing. Everyday, we are exposed to artificially sweetened diet foods and drinks that are reported to be healthier than foods sweetened with real sugar.

Are artificial sweeteners as healthy as food advertisers want us to believe? Unfortunately, data suggests that artificial sweeteners are just as harmful as real sugar. Studies suggest artificial sweeteners, even at dosages considered safe by the FDA, can be toxic to the body and brain, leading to increased inflammation and memory problems. Moreover, artificial sweeteners do not make you thinner. Just like sugar, they increase your craving for sweet foods, thus increasing intake of unhealthy and empty calories.

Aspartame is one of the most commonly used artificial sweeteners. It is commonly found in diet foods and drinks, such as diet soda, sugar-free gum, many sugar-free foods, and even prescription drugs and chewable vitamins.

Aspartame Effects on The Brain

Aspartame is associated with systemic inflammation, memory problems, migraine headaches, dementia, fibromyalgia, and even depression. After aspartame is ingested, it is metabolized into 3 isolates: Phenylalanine (50%). Aspartic Acid (40 %), Methanol (10 %).

Phenylalanine can cross the blood brain barrier (a special protective layer in the blood vessels surrounding the brain which provides extra protection for the highly sensitive brain). Phenylalanine crosses the blood brain barrier and causes severe changes in the production of dopamine and serotonin, important neurotransmitters that play a role in mood, sleep, and digestion.

Aspartic acid can also cross the blood brain barrier and bind to a special receptor in the brain called the NMDA receptor.

Excess binding to the NMDA receptor can lead to over-excitation of neurons, causing excitotoxicity. This leads to neuron death. Excess damage to neurons leads to cognitive and memory impairment.

Methanol is a toxic substance metabolized in the liver into formaldehyde (the chemical used to preserve dead bodies for autopsy). Formaldehyde is metabolized into formic acid which in excess can cause metabolic acidosis and tissue injury. The eyes are particularly sensitive to the toxic effects of methanol and can lead to blindness.

Aspartame's metabolites are also found in natural foods (i.e., milk, tomato juice, fruits). However, when found in natural foods, they are bound to other proteins and thus are released more slowly into the blood. When aspartame is consumed, it is rapidly absorbed into the blood stream. Therefore these toxic metabolites accumulate more rapidly in the blood. This rapid accumulation increases the risk for toxicity.

Even at dosages considered safe by the FDA (< 40 MB/KG), Aspartame consumption has been shown to be toxic to the brain. Its metabolites cause an increase in pro-inflammatory molecules in the brain. These pro-inflammatory molecules increase inflammation and also break down the protective blood brain barrier. Aspartame impairs learning and memory even at dosages considered save in humans.

A 2017 review of all the human and animal data on aspartame concluded that aspartame, even at recommended safe dosages might not be safe. The data suggested not only that aspartame is neurotoxic, but that aspartame also causes widespread damage to other organs in the body by causing anti-oxidant/oxidant imbalance, inducing oxidative stress (which is a hallmark of systemic inflammation), and causing tissue and organ injury. Ingestion of aspartame therefore likely contributes to systemic inflammation in people with diabetes and obesity, who already have high levels of systemic inflammation, and likely worsens overall health of people with these diseases.

Aspartame may not only worsen existing inflammation in diabetics and obese people, but also can induce systemic inflammation in healthy individuals. This brings about the hypothesis of whether aspartame is associated with the increasing rates of autoimmune disorders in developed nations where consumption of diet foods is high.

Sucralose, also known as Splenda

Sucralose, aka Splenda, is another artificial sweetener commonly used in diet foods and drinks. It was introduced in 1999 so there is less overall data about its effects compared to aspartame. While there is not much data on humans, rat studies show that sucralose can cause brain damage, especially to the hippocampus (a region in the brain important for memory formation). Sucralose also can decrease levels of good bacteria in the gut (good bacteria is important for proper gut health, immune system functioning, and for neurological and psychological health) Moreover, when sucralose is cooked at high temperatures, it breaks down and interacts with other ingredients, which can cause further harm. For example, sucralose can interact with glycerol which creates chloropropanol, a chemical that may increase cancer risk.

How can you avoid artificial sweeteners?

Now that you have been empowered with the knowledge about the harmful effects of artificial sweeteners, you are better equipped to make informed decisions about the substances you place in your body and that of your children's.

To avoid intake of toxic artificial sweeteners

1. Limit your intake of sweet food and drinks: Data suggests that both sugar and artificial sweeteners can increase systemic and brain inflammation. Sugar and artificial sweeteners also impair appetite mechanisms in the body (they can increase cravings for sweet foods) and thus cause weight gain.

The best way to avoid the harmful effects of artificial sweeteners and real sugar is to limit intake of sweet foods altogether.

2. Natural Sugar Substitutes: If it is difficult avoid sugars altogether, you can resort to natural sugar substitutes like monk fruit, stevia, xylitol. However even these three report through a few limited animal studies that stevia can cause unfavorable changes in dopamine and serotonin secretion in rat brains. Whenever you crave sugar, I recommend that you either eat a piece of fruit which has a lower glycemic index than any processed sweet food).

3. Read Food Labels Carefully. Foods that you never think would contain artificial sweeteners can contain aspartame or sucralose. Examples include diet/low sugar yogurt, salad dressing, whole wheat bread, condiments (i.e., ketchup), and sugar-free gum. Optimize your life by taking care of your brain.

Stroke and Dementia Risk Grows with Artificial Sweeteners. This information offers additional research results from the above and other artificial sweeteners. Diet sodas continue to gain negative attention and for good reason. A recent study found that consuming a daily can of sugar-free soda is associated with <u>higher risks of suffering a stroke or developing dementia</u>. Heavily sugared drinks already had a bad rap for causing a myriad of health issues such as weight gain, liver damage, kidney stones, diabetes, and heart disease.

Researchers found that drinking one diet soda a day is associated with a 2.96 times more likely chance of suffering an ischaemic stroke and a 2.89 times higher chance of developing Alzheimer's. While it would be irresponsible to imply that artificial sweeteners actually *cause* stroke or dementia (proving causation is very difficult in health studies) it is important to acknowledge the study's warning. There is a correlation between artificial sweeteners and the increased risk of dementia and stroke that's very concerning. It's certainly an added consideration that keeps me far away from diet sodas.

Sugar-Free Comes at a Cost

Artificial sweeteners have also been associated with health concerns besides stroke and dementia. A <u>2009 study</u> found that people who consumed diet drinks daily had a 67 percent higher risk for type 2 diabetes and a 36 percent higher risk of metabolic syndrome.

It's also been found, that artificial sweeteners can <u>dangerously impact your gut microbiome</u>. Another study suggests that artificial sweeteners favor bacteria that pull energy from food and convert it into fat. Meaning, If you are consuming zero calorie sweeteners specifically to cut down on weight gain, you might actually gain weight. Additionally, studies suggest that fake sugar can <u>induce glucose intolerance</u>, which can be a precursor of increased risk for liver and heart disease.

It's also been shown that artificial sweeteners can have a more potent taste and flood your sugar receptors. Meaning if you are regularly using artificial sweeteners you may find naturally sweet foods less appealing making it more difficult to satisfy your sweet craving. It can also contribute to making bitter foods such as vegetables taste downright disgusting. This can contribute to a vicious cycle of increased sugar intake, which can cause a cascading effect on your overall health.

If you are still using artificial sweeteners, I'm almost begging you to stop using these incredibly harmful substances. I promise there are healthier solutions to getting your sugar fix. I'll explain which natural sweeteners are best, but first let's look at some of the worst culprits in fake sugar.

The 6 Worst Artificial Sweeteners

Similar to sugar, your body can actually become addicted to artificial sweeteners, which is why it's a good idea to go ahead and rid your diet of any of these immediately. Some of the worst artificial sweeteners (and their common names) include:

Aspartame (NutraSweet and Equal) – Aspartame is about 200 times sweeter than table sugar. In a 2014 study published in the American Journal of Industrial Medicine, researchers called for "a re-evaluation of the current position of international regulatory agencies" with regard to aspartame. This study found that aspartame is a carcinogen and "must be considered an urgent matter of public health." Yikes!

Sucralose (Splenda) – Sucralose is about 600 times sweeter than table sugar and is well known for its propensity for being addictive. Multiple statements recently released by the Center for Science in the Public Interest have called for consumers to stop using Splenda pending more research due to the concerns that it may cause cancer.

Saccharin (Sweet 'N Low) – Saccharin is between 300 to 400 times sweeter than sugar and has no food energy. Many also notice it has a metallic aftertaste. Saccharin used to carry carcinogenic warnings but was _delisted in 2000 by the FDA_ due to a lack of evidence. Though the FDA has no limits on consumption, saccharin is still believed to contribute to health concerns and intake should be limited especially with _infants, children, and pregnant women._

Xylitol (Sorbitol, Maltitol, and other sugar alcohols ending in -itol) – Sugar alcohols aren't readily absorbed by your body and many find they are sensitive to xylitol. While xylitol is often added to breath mints and gum because it's known for its ability to kill bad bacteria of the mouth, it's also known for its gastrointestinal side effects. Gas, bloating, and diarrhea have all been linked to xylitol, which is why I recommend using xylitol in limited quantities. Be especially careful if you're pregnant or breastfeeding because not enough is known about xylitol. Please note: Xylitol is deadly to dogs, so keep your breath mints and sugar-free gum far away from your pup.

Acesulfame K (Sunett, Sweet One, ACE, ACE K) – ACE K is commonly found in sugar-free candy and has the fewest scientific studies when compared to other artificial sweeteners. Your body cannot break down ACE K and it may contain _methylene chloride_, which is known to cause side effects such as nausea, decreased alertness, headaches, irritability, and slow reaction times.

High fructose corn syrup – Technically, HFCS doesn't really fall under the "artificial" title because it's derived from corn. But the corn industry has tried to mislead the public into thinking this makes it a safe, natural alternative to sugar and that's simply not true. For the sake of calling HFCS exactly what it is – terrible for your health – I'm placing it on this list. HFCS has dangerous levels of fructose and studies have shown that fructose-sweetened beverages _increases the risk of metabolic and cardiovascular disorders._

The Best Natural Sweeteners

Every now and then, a sweet treat is in order, so let's look at the best natural sweeteners you can use instead of all that artificial garbage.

Raw honey – High in antioxidants, honey (especially local honey) is a great natural sugar option.

Palm sugar – Derived from palm sap, this sweetener contains trace amounts of phosphorous, iron, & vitamin C.

Blackstrap molasses – High in B vitamins, calcium, magnesium, iron, and manganese, blackstrap molasses is one of my favorite alternatives, especially in baking.

Medjool dates – Dates have health benefits such as high minerals and antioxidants but can be more time consuming to use.

Coconut sugar – This is a good alternative to brown sugar because they are similar in taste.

Maple syrup – Natural maple syrup is a better option than artificial sweeteners, but lower on my list of replacements.

There are delicious sweet options available to you – so there's really no need to load your body up with terrible artificial sweeteners that can make you sick. While the natural options are always better, it's important to watch your overall <u>sugar</u> intake.

Remember, high sugar intake has its own issues such as weight gain, kidney stones, liver damage, diabetes, and heart disease. Moderation is key in life and health, except for when it comes to artificial sweeteners. I think it's safe to say <u>ditching all artificial (chemical) sweeteners</u> is best.

foods consumed more calories than those that ate artificially sweetened foods. Both diabetes and obesity are considered independent risk factors for memory problems and several forms of dementia.

4. Artificial sugar substitutes mess with gut health. A 2018 found that six artificial sweeteners (aspartame, sucralose, saccharine, neotame, advantame, and acesulfame potassium-k) had toxic effects on gut bacteria. Compromised gut bacteria can lead to issues such as leaky gut, a condition in which the lining of the gut becomes excessively permeable. Leaky gut has been linked to the development of Alzheimer's disease and other dementias.

Sweeter Alternatives

If you want to avoid sugar and don't want the damage that comes from artificial sweeteners, here are two options.

Erythritol, a sugar alcohol that comes in crystals or powder form, is calorie-free and doesn't cause blood sugar or insulin levels to spike. (Note: Be aware that sugar alcohols, such as Xylitol and Maltitol, may cause GI distress.)

Stevia, a natural plant extract, is 200-300 times sweeter than sugar, but it does not impact blood sugar levels the way sugar does. Some evidence suggests stevia may stabilize blood sugar. However more research is needed. (Note: If you take medication for blood pressure or diabetes, talk to a healthcare provider before using stevia.)

It is critical for any changes in memory or cognitive function to be investigated. Research shows that changes in the brain from Alzheimer's disease can start decades before any symptoms arise. At this stage, there is imaging available to see what is happening in the brain as part of a comprehensive evaluation that also includes cognitive testing and a detailed look at the biological, psychological, social, and spiritual factors that may be contributing to memory issues.

Are Artificial Sweeteners Toxic to the Brain?

As sugar's harmful effects are becoming more widely acknowledged, the consumption of artificially sweetened foods and drinks is increasing. Everyday, we are exposed to artificially sweetened diet foods and drinks that are reported to be healthier than foods sweetened with real sugar.

Are artificial sweeteners as healthy as food advertisers want us to believe? Unfortunately, data suggests that artificial sweeteners are just as harmful as real sugar. Studies suggest artificial sweeteners, even at dosages considered safe by the FDA, can be toxic to the body and brain, leading to increased inflammation and memory problems. Moreover, artificial sweeteners do not make you thinner. Just like sugar, they increase your craving for sweet foods, thus increasing intake of unhealthy and empty calories.

Aspartame is one of the most commonly used artificial sweeteners. It is commonly found in diet foods and drinks, such as diet soda, sugar-free gum, many sugar-free foods, and even prescription drugs and chewable vitamins.

Aspartame Effects on The Brain

Aspartame is associated with systemic inflammation, memory problems, migraine headaches, dementia, fibromyalgia, and even depression. After aspartame is ingested, it is metabolized into 3 isolates: Phenylalanine (50%). Aspartic Acid (40 %), Methanol (10 %).

Phenylalanine can cross the blood brain barrier (a special protective layer in the blood vessels surrounding the brain which provides extra protection for the highly sensitive brain). Phenylalanine crosses the blood brain barrier and causes severe changes in the production of dopamine and serotonin, important neurotransmitters that play a role in mood, sleep, and digestion.

Aspartic acid can also cross the blood brain barrier and bind to a special receptor in the brain called the NMDA receptor. Excess binding to the NMDA receptor can lead to over-excitation of neurons, causing excitotoxicity. This leads to neuron death. Excess damage to neurons leads to cognitive and memory impairment.

Methanol is a toxic substance metabolized in the liver into formaldehyde (the chemical used to preserve dead bodies for autopsy). Formaldehyde is metabolized into formic acid which in excess can cause metabolic acidosis and tissue injury. The eyes are particularly sensitive to the toxic effects of methanol and can lead to blindness.

Aspartame's metabolites are also found in natural foods (i.e., milk, tomato juice, fruits). However, when found in natural foods, they are bound to other proteins and thus are released more slowly into the blood. When aspartame is consumed, it is rapidly absorbed into the blood stream. Therefore these toxic metabolites accumulate more rapidly in the blood. This rapid accumulation increases the risk for toxicity.

Even at dosages considered safe by the FDA (< 40 MB/KG), Aspartame consumption has been shown to be toxic to the brain. Its metabolites cause an increase in pro-inflammatory molecules in the brain. These pro-inflammatory molecules increase inflammation and also break down the protective blood brain barrier. Aspartame impairs learning and memory even at dosages considered save in humans.

A 2017 review of all the human and animal data on aspartame concluded that aspartame, even at recommended safe dosages might not be safe. The data suggested not only that aspartame is neurotoxic, but that aspartame also causes widespread damage to other organs in the body by causing anti-oxidant/oxidant imbalance, inducing oxidative stress (which is a hallmark of systemic inflammation), and causing tissue and organ injury. Ingestion of aspartame therefore likely contributes to systemic inflammation in people with diabetes and obesity, who already have high levels of systemic inflammation, and likely worsens overall health of people with these diseases.

Aspartame may not only worsen existing inflammation in diabetics and obese people, but also can induce systemic inflammation in healthy individuals. This brings about the hypothesis of whether aspartame is associated with the increasing rates of autoimmune disorders in developed nations where consumption of diet foods is high.

Sucralose, also known as Splenda

Sucralose, aka Splenda, is another artificial sweetener commonly used in diet foods and drinks. It was introduced in 1999 so there is less overall data about its effects compared to aspartame. While there is not much data on humans, rat studies show that sucralose can cause brain damage, especially to the hippocampus (a region in the brain important for memory formation). Sucralose also can decrease levels of good bacteria in the gut (good bacteria is important for proper gut health, immune system functioning, and for neurological and psychological health) Moreover, when sucralose is cooked at high temperatures, it breaks down and interacts with other ingredients, which can cause further harm. For example, sucralose can interact with glycerol which creates chloropropanol, a chemical that may increase cancer risk.

How can you avoid artificial sweeteners?

Now that you have been empowered with the knowledge about the harmful effects of artificial sweeteners, you are better equipped to make informed decisions about the substances you place in your body and that of your children's.

To avoid intake of toxic artificial sweeteners

2. Limit your intake of sweet food and drinks: Data suggests that both sugar and artificial sweeteners can increase systemic and brain inflammation. Sugar and artificial sweeteners also impair appetite mechanisms in the body (they can increase cravings for sweet foods) and thus cause weight gain.

The best way to avoid the harmful effects of artificial sweeteners and real sugar is to limit intake of sweet foods altogether.

2. Natural Sugar Substitutes: If it is difficult avoid sugars altogether, you can resort to natural sugar substitutes like monk fruit, stevia, xylitol. However even these three report through a few limited animal studies that stevia can cause unfavorable changes in dopamine and serotonin secretion in rat brains. Whenever you crave sugar, I recommend that you either eat a piece of fruit which has a lower glycemic index than any processed sweet food).

3. Read Food Labels Carefully. Foods that you never think would contain artificial sweeteners can contain aspartame or sucralose. Examples include diet/low sugar yogurt, salad dressing, whole wheat bread, condiments (i.e., ketchup), and sugar-free gum. Optimize your life by taking care of your brain.

Stroke and Dementia Risk Increase With Artificial Sweeteners

This information offers additional research results from the above and other artificial sweeteners. Diet sodas continue to gain negative attention and for good reason. A recent study found that consuming a daily can of sugar-free soda is associated with <u>higher risks of suffering a stroke or developing dementia</u>. Heavily sugared drinks already had a bad rap for causing a myriad of health issues such as weight gain, liver damage, kidney stones, diabetes, and heart disease.

Researchers found that drinking one diet soda a day is associated with a 2.96 times more likely chance of suffering an ischaemic stroke and a 2.89 times higher chance of developing Alzheimer's. While it would be irresponsible to imply that artificial sweeteners actually *cause* stroke or dementia (proving causation is very difficult in health studies) it is important to acknowledge the study's warning. There is a correlation between artificial sweeteners and the increased risk of dementia and stroke that's very concerning. It's certainly an added consideration that keeps me far away from diet sodas.

Sugar-Free Comes at a Cost

Artificial sweeteners have also been associated with health concerns besides stroke and dementia. A <u>2009 study</u> found that people who consumed diet drinks daily had a 67 percent higher risk for type 2 diabetes and a 36 percent higher risk of metabolic syndrome.

It's also been found, that artificial sweeteners can <u>dangerously impact your gut microbiome</u>. Another study suggests that artificial sweeteners favor bacteria that pull energy from food and convert it into fat. Meaning, If you are consuming zero calorie sweeteners specifically to cut down on weight gain, you might actually gain weight. Additionally, studies suggest that fake sugar can <u>induce glucose intolerance</u>, which can be a precursor of increased risk for liver and heart disease.

It's also been shown that artificial sweeteners can have a more potent taste and flood your sugar receptors. Meaning if you are regularly using artificial sweeteners you may find naturally sweet foods less appealing making it more difficult to satisfy your sweet craving. It can also contribute to making bitter foods such as vegetables taste downright disgusting. This can contribute to a vicious cycle of increased sugar intake, which can cause a cascading effect on your overall health.

If you are still using artificial sweeteners, I'm almost begging you to stop using these incredibly harmful substances. I promise there are healthier solutions to getting your sugar fix. I'll explain which natural sweeteners are best, but first let's look at some of the worst culprits in fake sugar.

The 6 Worst Artificial Sweeteners

Similar to sugar, your body can actually become addicted to artificial sweeteners, which is why it's a good idea to go ahead and rid your diet of any of these immediately. Some of the worst artificial sweeteners (and their common names) include:

<u>Aspartame</u> (NutraSweet and Equal) – Aspartame is about 200 times sweeter than table sugar. In a <u>2014 study published in the American Journal of Industrial Medicine</u>, researchers called for "a re-evaluation of the current position of international regulatory agencies" with regard to aspartame. This study found that aspartame is a carcinogen and "must be considered an urgent matter of public health." Yikes!

Sucralose (Splenda) – Sucralose is about 600 times sweeter than table sugar and is well known for its propensity for being addictive. Multiple statements recently released by the <u>Center for Science in the Public Interest</u> have called for consumers to stop using Splenda pending more research due to the concerns that it may cause cancer.

Saccharin (Sweet 'N Low) – Saccharin is between 300 to 400 times sweeter than sugar and has no food energy. Many also notice it has a metallic aftertaste. Saccharin used to carry carcinogenic warnings but was <u>delisted in 2000 by the FDA</u> due to a lack of evidence. Though the FDA has no limits on consumption, saccharin is still believed to contribute to health concerns and intake should be limited especially with <u>infants, children, and pregnant women</u>.

<u>Xylitol</u> (Sorbitol, Maltitol, and other sugar alcohols ending in -itol) – Sugar alcohols aren't readily absorbed by your body and many find they are sensitive to xylitol. While xylitol is often added to breath mints and gum because it's known for its ability to kill bad bacteria of the mouth, it's also known for its gastrointestinal side effects. Gas, bloating, and diarrhea have all been linked to xylitol, which is why I recommend using xylitol in limited quantities. Be especially careful if you're pregnant or

breastfeeding because not enough is known about xylitol. Please note: Xylitol is deadly to dogs, so keep your breath mints and sugar-free gum far away from your pup.

Acesulfame K (Sunett, Sweet One, ACE, ACE K) – ACE K is commonly found in sugar-free candy and has the fewest scientific studies when compared to other artificial sweeteners. Your body cannot break down ACE K and it may contain methylene chloride, which is known to cause side effects such as nausea, decreased alertness, headaches, irritability, and slow reaction times.

High fructose corn syrup – Technically, HFCS doesn't really fall under the "artificial" title because it's derived from corn. But the corn industry has tried to mislead the public into thinking this makes it a safe, natural alternative to sugar and that's simply not true. For the sake of calling HFCS exactly what it is – terrible for your health – I'm placing it on this list. HFCS has dangerous levels of fructose and studies have shown that fructose-sweetened beverages increases the risk of metabolic and cardiovascular disorders.

The Best Natural Sweeteners

Every now and then, a sweet treat is in order, so let's look at the best natural sweeteners you can use instead of all that artificial garbage.

Raw honey – High in antioxidants, honey (especially local honey) is a great natural sugar option.

Palm sugar – Derived from palm sap, this sweetener contains trace amounts of phosphorous, iron, & vitamin C.

Blackstrap molasses – High in B vitamins, calcium, magnesium, iron, and manganese, blackstrap molasses is one of my favorite alternatives, especially in baking.

Medjool dates – Dates have health benefits such as high minerals and antioxidants but can be more time consuming to use.

Coconut sugar – This is a good alternative to brown sugar because they are similar in taste.

Maple syrup – Natural maple syrup is a better option than artificial sweeteners, but lower on my list of replacements.

There are delicious sweet options available to you – so there's really no need to load your body up with terrible artificial sweeteners that can make you sick. While the natural options are always better, it's important to watch your overall _sugar_ intake.

Remember, high sugar intake has its own issues such as weight gain, kidney stones, liver damage, diabetes, and heart disease. Moderation is key in life and health, except for when it comes to artificial sweeteners. I think it's safe to say <u>ditching all artificial (chemical) sweeteners</u> is best.

Pure, White and Deadly – How Sugar is killing us

John Yudkin (1910 - 1995) was a British physiologist and nutritionist. He became internationally famous with his book *"Pure, White and Deadly"* first published in 1972, as one of the first scientists to claim that sugar was a major cause of obesity and heart disease.

In the 1960s, Dr. John Yudkin, a UK nutritionist, was conducting research into the deleterious effects of sugar. In those days to the present nutritional orthodoxy held that the arch dietary villain was saturated fat. Low-fat diets became the mantra of nutrition science and public health dietary recommendations.

In 1972, he published Pure, White and Deadly in which he outlined the results of his scientific findings showing that sugar and carbohydrates – not fat — raised blood levels of triglycerides increased the risk for heart disease in rodents, chickens, rabbits, pigs and students. Sugar also raised insulin levels, linking it directly to type-2 diabetes.

Dr. Yudkin noted that we had been eating substances like butter for centuries, while sugar, had, up until the 1850s, been something of a rare treat for most people. "If only a small fraction of what we know about the effects of sugar were to be revealed in relation to any other material used as a food additive," he wrote, "that material would promptly be banned."

Clearly, Dr. Yudkin and the book – which sold well – posed a threat to the processed food industry which has been pumping sugar into most processed foods, including baby food. The World Sugar Research Organization described the book as "science fiction."

A concerted vilification campaign was orchestrated by industry and several prominent nutritionists who sought to destroy his reputation. Ancel Keys was the most vicious vocal character assassin who succeeded in marginalizing and discrediting Dr. Yudkin, whose career never recovered. He died, in 1995, a disappointed, largely forgotten man for the next 50 years, as was his book.

In 2009, Dr. Yudkin's scientific work finally was acknowledged as "prophetic" and groundbreaking by Dr. Robert Lustig, a professor of pediatric endocrinology at the University of California, who specializes in treating childhood obesity, who brought Dr. Yudkin's work to light.

"Everything this man said in 1972 was the God's honest truth and if you want to read a true prophecy you find this book. I'm telling you every single thing this guy said has come to pass. I'm in awe and Science took a disastrous detour in ignoring Dr. Yudkins work. It was to the detriment of the health of millions.

Dr. Yudkin's book has been republished and gives full details on how sugar is dangerous to our health. You are welcome to search for used and new versions on the internet. No details of that insightful book are here but I highly recommend it to better understand why we are growing into a sick and overweight population with the average life span actually shortening rather than improving – even before the Coronavirus Pandemic.

The Best 15 Alkaline Foods on the Planet

Follows are foods that will help improve your natural immunity through their vitamins and minerals contained within.

1. Spinach

Spinach can eliminate free radicals, improve your memory, and keep your heart strong by being rich in antioxidants. Furthermore, it can stimulate your brain function. It is low in fat and cholesterol, it has vitamins A, C, K, B6, and contains magnesium, potassium, calcium, zinc, iron, and niacin.

2. Lemons

The lemon juice can reduce the risk of stroke, and it can also help treat kidney stones. Another positive side to the lemon is that it helps fight cancer, prevent constipation and high blood pressure. It has vitamins E, A, C, B6, and many important minerals like zinc, calcium, potassium, copper, and riboflavin.

3. Quinoa

It can help with the cholesterol and blood sugar level in your body. It is the food that is the richest in proteins and compared to other grains it has twice the amount of fiber. Moreover, quinoa is rich in manganese, magnesium, riboflavin, lysine and iron.

4. Swiss Chard

The Swiss chard helps with blood sugar, and improves the health of your heart and your blood circulation. It helps the body stay away from viruses, harmful bacteria, and free radicals. Also, it is the best source of alkali from all foods known to us.

5. Buckwheat

This wheat is nothing like the regular one, since it can improve your heart health, prevent diabetes, and boost your energy levels. It keeps your body warm, so it's a perfect meal for the winter's cold days. In addition, buckwheat is a great source of vitamins, iron, and protein.

6. Melon

The melon will clear the toxins from your body and at the same time keep you hydrated. What makes it a top alkaline food is its pH value that is around 8,5. The water content of this fruit is very high, and that is why it is a good example of an alkaline food.

7. Olive oil

Olive oil regulates the blood sugar levels and reduces the risk of heart disease. It is rich in vitamin E, monounsaturated fatty acids, and antioxidants. So, we recommend adding it to your diet.

8. Bananas

If you want to lose weight you better add bananas to your daily diet. This fruit balances the blood sugar levels, protects the heart and improves the digestion. In addition, it is rich in fiber and nutrients like potassium, manganese, B vitamins, and magnesium.

9. Flaxseed

These seeds keep the heart healthy, help control the hot flashes in menopause and reduce inflammations. The flaxseed is considered as a top alkaline food since it is rich in fiber, antioxidants and vitamin E. Therefore, we recommend you use it every day. You can grind the flaxseed and add it to almost any meal.

10. Cauliflower

It boosts the heart health and has anti-inflammatory properties. One serving of this vegetable provides 77 percent of the daily requirement of vitamin C. Moreover, cauliflower is abundant in riboflavin, potassium, magnesium, vitamin K, thiamin, and manganese.

11. Avocados

Avocados help the absorption of nutrients from vegetables and fruits, control the levels of cholesterol and make your heart stronger. You can reap the benefits of this super-food by consuming even a bowl of guacamole. What's more, the avocado contains fiber, nutrients, and monounsaturated fatty acids.

12. Grapes

They help reduce anxiety and hypertension. This fruit reduces the risk of lung, prostate, colon, esophageal, pancreatic, endometrial, and mouth cancer, due to its polyphenols (antioxidants).

13. Carrots

Carrots improve your thought process and your eyesight due to their beta-carotene content (a group of pigments) which protect you against free radical damage. They are high in vitamin K, C, A, B8, iron, potassium, and fiber.

14. Broccoli

This vegetable improves the blood circulation due to its high amounts of iron. It keeps the heart healthy, improves the health of bones, and reduces the levels of cholesterol. What's more, broccoli is also a powerful antioxidant which helps fight cancer. It is rich in copper, fiber, potassium and vitamin K, B6, C, and E.

15. Berries

Berries improve the skin and are good food to slow down the aging process. They help with chronic health disorders, and keep a sharp memory as you grow old.

Suggested Shopping List:

Proteins: Low-fat milk, eggs, tinned tuna or sardines, lean beef, chicken or soya mince, chicken portions or breasts

Plant proteins: All types of dry beans, soya beans, lentils and chickpeas

Healthy starch: Rolled oats, brown rice, pearled barley or seeded health bread

Fruit and vegetables: Seasonal fruit, bananas, lemons, tinned and fresh tomatoes, cucumber, carrots, onions, gem squash, cabbage, butternut and spinach

Fats: Light mayonnaise, peanut butter, olive or canola oil

Other: Herbs and spices, salt and pepper, tea and coffee

Where Our Nutrients Come From

The most essential mineral elements of the body composition, in order of their apparent importance, are iodine, copper, calcium, phosphorus, manganese, sodium, potassium, magnesium, chlorine, and sulfur. All but the first of these, iodine, which is a native of the sea, have their source in the soil.

We would naturally suppose that when we eat products of the soil we should secure an ample supply of them. That is what Nature intended. But Nature did not foresee that man would remove the trees and other growth, allowing the rains to erode the soil, leaching out the essential minerals and, my means of our creeks and rivers, carrying them down to the sea. The result has been mineral-starved soils, in turn producing mineral-starved foods. The obvious result is that humans now depend upon these mineral-starved foods for our supply of minerals and are literally starving in the midst of plenty.

It is easy to know when one is hungry for sweets, starches, or fats. The body sends out distress signals almost immediately and, if we are in normal health, our appetite tells us what is needed.

Once we learn to know them, the signs of mineral hunger are quite as definite and the results, if our body's SOS it long ignored, are far more serious.

There have developed within the last few generations, especially here in the United States, where food is most abundant and the average person eats most generously a whole series of deficiency diseases. It is recognized that each of these diseases is due to a lack of vital elements in the diet, and the essentials most often lacking are the essential minerals. The thyroid requires iodine. The parathyroid requires cobalt and nickel. The adrenal glands require magnesium. The pancreas requires cobalt and nickel. The anterior pituitary gland needs manganese. The posterior pituitary needs chlorine. The gonads require iron.

Iron enters directly into the construction of the hemoglobin of red corpuscles, which are the oxygen carriers of our blood. Anemia is a deficiency disease which may develop if there is an insufficient supply of iron in the blood. Unfortunately the human body cannot store up much iron, to it is necessary to replenish the supply regularly.

As our soils become more impoverished, the seas become richer in those minerals. However, we find an ocean plant whose botanical name is Macrocystis pyrifera and which is commonly called *kelp*. It is often referred to as a sea vegetable and serves well as a food supplement.

Kelp grows in great abundance off the California coast. It flourishes best at a depth of six to ten fathoms and is found only where the ocean bottom is rocky. It has no roots but is anchored to the rocks by tough ropelike cables and derives its nourishment entirely from the water. It is one of the largest plants in existence, often growing as much as fifty feet in a single year. Each plant consists of a trunk or stem, lined on either side with large single lanceolate leaves. The leaves occur in files of six or eight or more, the files alternating, each leaf supported by a buoy or floater at its point of contact with the trunk of the plant. Each leaf is finely but irregularly corrugated, is bordered with a single row of short, soft spines, and is olive brown in color.

Biochemistry teaches us that plants are the only organisms that can manufacture food, and that the essential food elements man receives from the flesh of animals come originally from plants. As every raw material essential for plant life is right at hand, the seaweeds such as kelp are naturally rich in the food elements required by man and other forms of animal life. The minerals it absorbs from the water in such abundance are present in an organic colloidal state, readily usable, and directly transferrable to the human body.

The Importance of Iodine

Folk medicine in Vermont is interested in three R's – Resistance, Repair, and Recovery. First the individual asks himself whether his resistance to disease is as it should be. Next, is he able to repair tissue injury due to accident should it occur? Finally, if sickness should occur, is his body able to bring about recovery?

Iodine is necessary for the thyroid gland's proper performance of its work. All the blood in the body passes through the thyroid gland every 17 minutes. Strong, virulent germs are rendered weaker during their passage through the thyroid gland. With each 17 minutes that rolls around they are made still weaker until finally they are killed *if* the gland has it normal supply of Iodine.

This gland also rebuilds energy and endurance in the individual. Iodine also relieves nervous tension. When nervous tension runs high there is irritability and difficulty in sleeping well at night. The body is continually on a combat basis, organized for fight and flight. Iodine can relax the body and enable it to organize for peace and quiet. Iodine also relates to clear thinking.

One cause for the thyroid to lose Iodine is sodium chloride or "Table Salt".

Here are three ways to bring up the iodine content when needed:

1.   Eat foods that are particularly high in iodine: Radishes, asparagus, carrots, tomatoes, spinach, rhubarb, potatoes, peas, strawberries, mushrooms, lettuce, bananas, cabbage, egg yolk and onions contain iodine.
2.   You may also paint a small area of the body with tincture of Iodine which is then absorbed through the skin.
3.   Preparations known to be rich in iodine include Cod-liver oil, Lugol's solution of iodine, and kelp tablets.

One executive's answer to keep his blood on the thin, free-flowing side is by omitting wheat foods, wheat cereals, white sugar, and citrus fruits and fruit juices. The reasoning is because in most people, those foods change the normal acid reaction of the urine to alkaline – a signal that the blood is thicker than it should be causing more work on the heart.

Therefore the man omits and replaces the unwise foods with rye and corn foods and cereals. Instead of white sugar he uses honey. In place of citrus foods and juices, he may use apple, grape, or cranberry juice.

At lunchtime he takes two teaspoonfuls of apple cider vinegar and two teaspoonfuls of honey in a glass of water. In this way he obtains acid taken up from the soil by fruit, berries, edible leaves, and roots, and the energy from the sun which exists in honey. This is a prime pick-up drink.

Observations have been made in the use of Corn oils such as Mazola Oil. One tablespoon of corn oil at one or all three meals each day had been helpful in hay fever, asthma, and migraine, because it helps in keeping the urine on the acid side. Corn oil is of value in shifting the body chemistry from alkaline to acid.

If the margins of the eyelids are scaly and granulated, one tablespoonful of corn oil by mouth at breakfast, and again at the evening meal, will, within one month's time, generally cure the condition. The same treatment for eczema is to remove scales leaving the skin soft and pliable.

Feel free to order a copy of the book "Vermont Folk Medicine" by D. C. Jarvis, M.D. with the subtitle: "A famous doctor's guide to folk medicine practices of Vermont – the nature secrets of honey, apple cider vinegar, and foods for health." Much of the 191 page book also includes tips for livestock care.

These tips may very well protect all of us from the threat of the coronavirus currently assaulting the northern hemisphere. March 5, 2020.

Companion books linked to "Natural Virus Protection"
Recommended reading for more detailed information.

Pure, White and Deadly, by John Yudkin
How sugar is killing us and what we can do to stop it.
In his 1972 book, Dr. John Yudkin, a United Kingdom nutritionist, conducted detailed research into the deleterious effects of sugar. His studies showed that sugar and other refined carbohydrates like sugar-sweetened beverages, pastries, white bread, white pasta, white rice and others were more dangerous even than fat intake for adverse effects on the human body and could weaken natural immunities to disease and other disorders.

Vermont Folk Medicine by Dr. D.C. Jarvis
A famous doctor's 1958 guide to folk medicine practices on the nature of Honey and Apple Cider Vinegar to improve your overall health. Dr. Jarvis' purpose is to bring knowledge and understanding of the capability and uses of folk medicine for improving natural body immunity to be free of physical impairment and weakness from disease and virus infections.

These two doctor's prophetic understanding of the natural immunity found in the human body show how humans are easily led through advertising to eat foods for taste rather than for health. However you do not have to give up your favorite foods if you follow the recommendations in this book to limit or to add some simple additives to return to good health and natural immunity to diseases.

About the Editor

Marlys J. Waters was born and raised on a farm near Nemaha, Iowa. After graduating from Crestland Community School (Early and Nemaha) in 1963, she attended Iowa State University and Drake University, and worked thirty years in the Des Moines area.

Marlys returned to her hometown of Nemaha in 1993 to care for her parents where she started "Power of the Pen Publishing. She also writes books and compiles music books for resale.

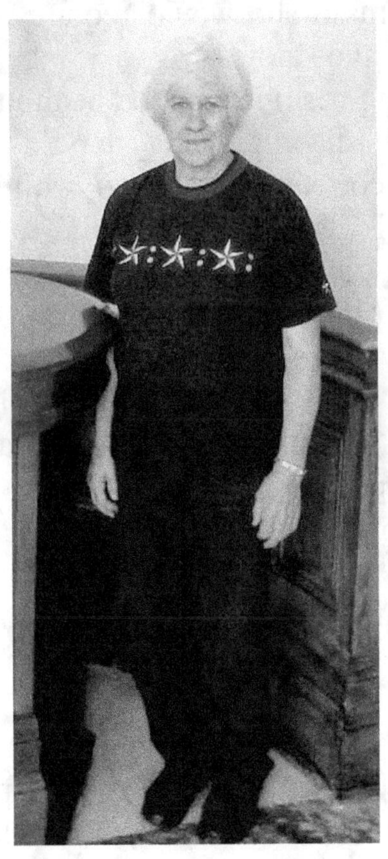

Note: Author Marlys J. Waters gave up common sugar and candy at age 50, and all highly processed sugars at age 65. She lost 50 pounds, and has not needed a doctor's care for over 25 years – no colds, no flu, no coughing, and has retained an active lifestyle at age 74.

She can still walk long distances with no dizzy spells, light knee pain that disappears when resting, and no skin disorders.

Marlys also uses a serving of spinach (cooked, canned, or raw) daily from a tip she learned when she was working full time and taking college classes in her 30s. She had read that spinach would help keep away infections and virus, and would also revitalize her system so she would require less sleep and have more time for work and studies.

She is now sharing her tips on good health to assist others who are struggling with disorders that the doctors are unable to understand and to correct. Tips found within should also help build your natural immunity to aid from contracting the Coronavirus. If you have a mild case like those who have tested positive but after 18 days in isolation never had any of symptoms, you survived!

Mild symptoms may not require hospitalization but the following severe symptoms should be treated at a hospital. Symptoms may appear 2-14 days after exposure to the virus. People with these mild symptoms may have COVID-19:

Fever or chills, cough, shortness of breath or difficulty breathing, fatigue, muscle or body aches, headache, new loss of taste or smell, sore throat, congestion or runny nose, nausea or vomiting, diarrhea.

If someone is showing these severe signs, seek emergency medical care: Trouble breathing, Persistent pain or pressure in the chest, New confusion, Inability to wake or stay awake, Bluish lips or face - Call your medical provider immediately..

9 781716 687341